MW01686788

Book Design by Rick Schank, Purple Couch Creative

Human Anatomy Illustrations © Marjorie Leggitt

Printed in Canada

ISBN: 979-8-9871648-0-8 (paperback)

Environmental Benefits Statement

By using paper made with 100% post-consumer recycled content, the following resources have been saved.

trees	water	energy	solid waste	greenhouse gases
16	1,250	6.9	56.3	7,016
fully grown	gallons	million BTU	pounds	pounds

Environmental impact estimates were made using the Environmental Paper Network Paper Calculator Version 4.0
For more information visit www.papercalculator.org
FSC® is not responsible for any calculations on saving resources by choosing this paper

FSC www.fsc.org RECYCLED Paper made from recycled material FSC® C014956

zero 100% carbon neutral by Hemlock Printers www.hemlock.com/zero

“

The payoffs of courage and effort to create change aren’t always immediately obvious, but they work as a mighty tectonic force that can shift the future in fundamental ways.

– Yvon Chouinard, Patagonia

”

TABLE OF CONTENTS

DEAR ATHLETE

DEAR ATHLETE,

We share the love of sport. We share the love of winning or striving to win and of being considered the best. We share the hours of repeated practice—the training that's required to build muscle memory and reach excellence. Prior to competing, we share the nerves so raw they feel as if they've broken through our bodies to the outside in their fight for more oxygen. We share life in a bubble to do what we do.

I understand the full spectrum of athleticism, inside and out. My life has been devoted to being an athlete, whether I'm training and competing at the world-class level, enjoying a recreational activity, or working with others as their sports psychologist or coach. In my younger years, I was a swimmer and springboard diver. In college, I competed on both nordic and alpine ski teams and played single and doubles tennis starting on the varsity team. Post-college, living on my own in California, I discovered a deep love of cycling, one that had been growing since my twin sister and I rode hundreds of miles starting at age 14 when our dad bought us identical Peugeot ten-speeds. I fortuitously found myself in a relationship with Joe Breeze, the man who created the first modern mountain bike. Together, we rode both road and mountain bikes, we founded NORBA—National Off Road Bicycling Association—a movement that introduced the mountain bike to the world, and we then raced at all of the NORBA-sanctioned mountain bike races. Carefully, we outlined essential rules for mountain biking to create guidance and harmony sharing trails with hikers, runners, equestrians, and others. At the time, we had no idea that our efforts would catapult one of the world's most loved sports into existence and manifest what is today a multi-billion dollar global industry.

Through mountain bike racing, I met my husband and together we raised our daughters within the world of sport—mountain biking, road cycling, nordic and alpine skiing, snow-shoeing, hiking, tennis, swimming, kayaking, stand-up paddling, and more. At age 42, I immersed myself into XTERRA off-road triathlons, while nurturing my kids' growing passion for ski racing. Over the next 20 years I treasured being involved in my daughters' athletic pursuits, while expanding my own legacy of training, traveling, and racing around the world. Simultaneously, my career as a sports psychologist, public speaker, and author blossomed.

In late 2010, while at the top of my game, something shocking happened. As I was packing my bags for the XTERRA European Championships in Switzerland, I climbed high into my closet to get a gift for the race director and slipped, falling hard and fracturing both of my heels. Suddenly, a wildly active lifestyle and my competitive athletic world felt beyond reach. But as it turned out, I needed this moment—the universe had other ideas for me.

With my physical recovery came personal reflection. I began to ask difficult questions about my goodness, worth, and impact on the world. Did such focused intensity as an athlete help those around me or just help me? I felt the person I was known to be—a devoted mother, champion of sport, mentor, and inspiration to others—had fallen short. I now saw myself as someone who was too singularly focused, living in a self-absorbed and self-indulgent bubble. I was embarrassed and ashamed because I knew better. My heels were broken and now my heart as well.

This self-reflection led me to an important

realization: that I can be a champion in sport endlessly preparing for challenges in swim-bike-run, while also caring about challenges facing humanity and the environment. It was the first time the concept of whole champion came to me. It came to me in a crystal clear way, that "whole" is what is missing in the cache of "champion."

For me, competing in sport will always be an adrenaline rush, and it's empowering to stand on a podium and receive a medal. I love winning, but I now deeply value the winning principles of caring about others and using my talents, drive, and dedication to make a positive difference for humanity and our damaged environment. I whispered to my family one night at dinner from my wheelchair, "Hey guys, I want to be a whole champion."

Armed with new understanding and desire to make a difference in the world, I

To uncover your true potential you must first find your own limits and then you have to have the courage to blow past them.

– Picabo Street

founded the Whole Champion Foundation in 2016. I felt it was time to care not only about myself, but also about the greater whole. To do this, I wanted to get other athletes, other role models, and key influencers on board.

I expanded my winning race mantra of "Yes I can" to something more expansive and meaningful: "Yes I can...inspire people to value their own and others' well-being, to live by kindness and inclusiveness, and to take a stand for equality, justice, and the environment."

I redefined whole and champion and connected the two words to become a new global understanding, a concept that everyone can have an impact. **I define "whole" as a conscious mindset where there is little separation between personal, social, and environmental responsibility. "Champion" is every individual who steps up and takes action towards a meaningful cause.**

Regardless of age, gender, or background, we each have the power to make a difference, to champion positive change one person, one cause, one day at a time.

As athletes, we aspire to specific goals through dedication, practice, and commitment to excellence. We have great respect for our bodies. We work endlessly on our physical, mental, and spiritual strengths. But as athletes today, there is much more to consider. It's one thing to be a person who earns titles, trophies, and steps up to the podium and another thing to be someone who also steps up to help the greater whole. **This book is for the best role model I know—you. Now is the time to integrate your personal care with purpose beyond yourself. My message for you can be boiled down to these few words: today it is vitally important that there is little separation between personal, social, and environmental responsibility.**

You, your family, coaches, friends, and whole community will benefit when you intentionally and consciously leverage your athletic aspirations to include care of challenges near and far. As a strong and inspiring athlete, you possess an ideal platform to influence change for a better world. I believe that a Whole Athlete offers a special way to make the whole world better. This book delves into how to do that.

Thank you for considering the enormous potential to give and explore your positive life as an athlete, a role model, and a leader for a better world.

Sport has the power to change the world. It has the power to inspire. It has the power to unite people in a way that little else does.

– Nelson Mandela

GLOBAL RESPONSIBILITY

PRACTICING LITTLE SEPARATION BETWEEN PERSONAL, SOCIAL, AND ENVIRONMENTAL RESPONSIBILITY

CHOOSING TO BE A WHOLE ATHLETE MEANS caring about yourself, your fellow humans, plants and animals, and our planet that is in crisis. Barack Obama said, "Now is the time for all of us to take our share of responsibility for a global response to global challenges." I agree.

Being a Whole Athlete means adding greater consciousness and care to the stellar person you already are. It means today and every day you understand the importance and practice of having awareness and taking care of your best self and the world outside yourself. It means you are fueled by caring for your own well-being and enhancing your own athletic performance, *and* you make a positive difference elsewhere. It means you thrive on and share a fortified diet of compassion, care, and love, knowing these are the necessities of life for one and all. The truth is, without these essential principles, humanity cannot survive. At its essence, this attitude and understanding is how we embrace global responsibility.

To get to the heart of global responsibility and to fully understand what little separation means, let's unpack its pieces—personal, social, and environmental responsibility.

> **So, we can't save the world by playing by the rules, because the rules have to be changed. Everything needs to change and it has to start today.**
>
> – Greta Thunberg

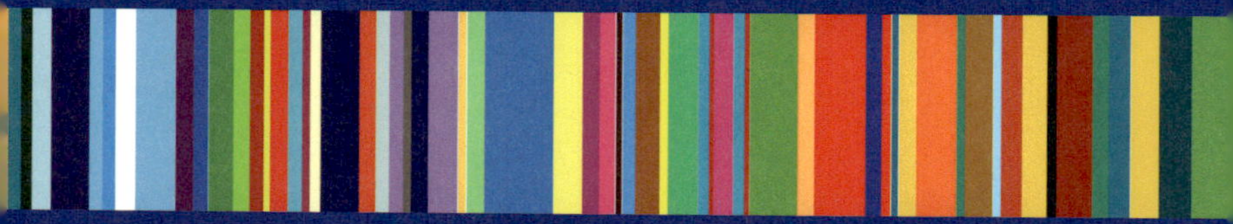

PERSONAL RESPONSIBILITY

CULTIVATING PHYSICAL, MENTAL, AND EMOTIONAL WELL-BEING AS A WHOLE ATHLETE

PERSONAL
RESPONSIBILITY

LOOKS
LIKE THIS

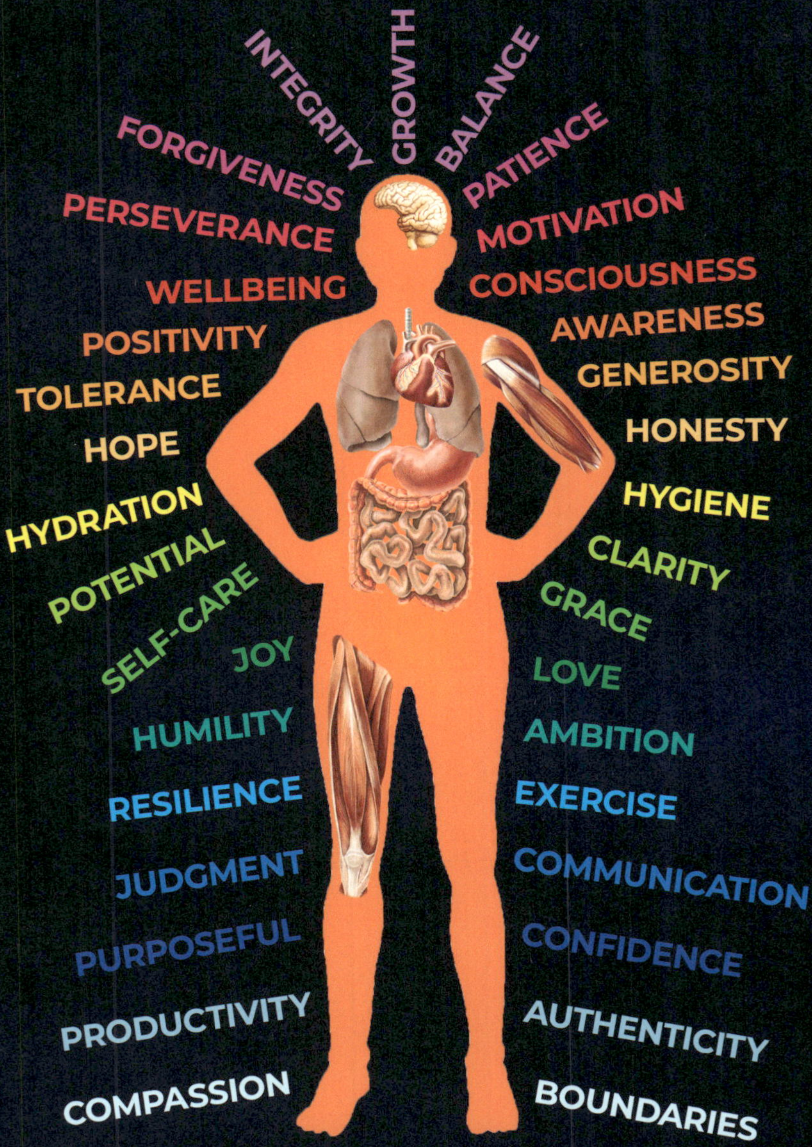
INTEGRITY
GROWTH
BALANCE
FORGIVENESS
PATIENCE
PERSEVERANCE
MOTIVATION
WELLBEING
CONSCIOUSNESS
POSITIVITY
AWARENESS
TOLERANCE
GENEROSITY
HOPE
HONESTY
HYDRATION
HYGIENE
POTENTIAL
CLARITY
SELF-CARE
GRACE
JOY
LOVE
HUMILITY
AMBITION
RESILIENCE
EXERCISE
JUDGMENT
COMMUNICATION
PURPOSEFUL
CONFIDENCE
PRODUCTIVITY
AUTHENTICITY
COMPASSION
BOUNDARIES

ATHLETES ARE TYPICALLY TUNNEL-VISIONED to hone skills and grow the drive to win. Cultivating personal will, focus, and dedication is personal responsibility, and a given for athletes. This meaning of personal responsibility is understood and so is staying isolated by this. A Whole Athlete isn't isolated. A Whole Athlete is empowered and effective when their intensified life force is applied to sport and things greater than their sport. A Whole Athlete approaches athletic challenges and triumphs while extending themselves to other important challenges and triumphs.

GLOBAL IS THE NEW PERSONAL RESPONSIBILITY

Act Locally, Think Globally

For a Whole Athlete, personal responsibility is complex, nuanced, and individual. As an athlete, you have found personal success by taking personal responsibility. You are exceptionally fit, and you care about your overall health. You have a life force that serves you well. Chances are you are also energized and productive at school or work or at managing your home and family.

Personal responsibility is the first step towards embodying the values and lifestyle of a whole person. It is caring for yourself, holding yourself accountable, practicing self-compassion and self-respect. For a Whole Athlete, it is understanding the power of being a whole person, which also includes respecting your human and personal limits and boundaries and choices that are aligned with living with balance and integrity. It is not about striving for absolute perfection; rather, it's about conscious effort and dedication to 'do life' to the best of your abilities. **Personal responsibility is caring deeply about the well-being of your body, mind, and spirit.**

Take a moment to reflect on yourself. You are a human with needs. You are also an exceptional athlete with focused intentions and a cultivated skill set. Again, you take personal responsibility for this. As a Whole Athlete, you are aware that there may be parts of yourself needing extra attention. An athlete who cultivates a strong heart, along with a well-conditioned body, most often finds success. **A Whole Athlete discovers ways to make their voice and actions as strong as their body.**

For athletes, "success" can mean any number of things: making it to the podium, breaking a personal record, mastering a new technique, a personal honoring of what it took to reach your level of excellence, overcoming a challenge, and conquering all obstacles.

We strive to win because it equates to success. We instantly feel proud and confident, and being in the spotlight feels magical. But the truth is, winning and the rush of confidence and success can sometimes feel fleeting. We shine for a moment and then it's done. Some athletes feel an emotional letdown...until they compete again. I believe it is the athlete who expands their efforts and applies their skill sets and intentions to parts of life beyond their sport, who experiences sustained success.

PERSONAL RESPONSIBILITY BUILDS EQUANIMITY

Equanimity is the signature attribute of a Whole Athlete. It is inner and outer strength.

> **With great power comes great responsibility.**
>
> **– Spiderman's motto**

It comes from having compassion, focus, confidence, and appreciation of your special brilliance. It is personal empowerment. With equinimity, you understand that life is about care, awareness, and choices. You not only care about high performance, but also expansion, exploration, discovery, life-long learning, and giving. You also understand the benefit of being part of the greater whole. This is the ultimate win!

PHYSICAL HEALTH

Balancing momentum, peak performance, and physical limitations through hydration • rest • nutrition

For an athlete, the body is the essential tool. The body can be pushed in many ways and in many directions, but should never be forced to go beyond its essential limitations. The body is a sacred vessel that affords extraordinary physical possibilities and life experiences when treated with respect, kindness, and balance.

As an ambitious athlete whose physical well-being is of the highest importance, your performance depends upon care of the highest order.

These essential elements support physical well-being for every athlete:

Hydration:

Hydration is paramount for all athletes. **Water is the single most important nutrient of life.** Without water, metabolic and physiological processes within the body cannot occur. All biochemical reactions in the body require water. The human body is approximately 70% water, our brain tissue is approximately 75% water, and our blood is roughly 83% water. Water transports nutrients; stimulates digestion; eliminates waste and flushes out toxins; regulates body temperature; lowers cortisol; lubricates your spine, bones, joints, muscles; aids in fat loss and boosts metabolism; and supports brain function, including memory and cognitive performance. We can live for weeks without food, but we can only live for a few days without water. Performance cannot be sustained without being properly hydrated!

Best Practices:

- Always bring a reusable water bottle
- Set a water goal for the day
- Flavor water with fruits, vegetables, and juices
- Use alarms or notifications as reminders to drink water

Rest:

For survival, **sleep is like air, water, and food.** For performance, rest is a fundamental biological component to optimize ambitious goals and overall well-being. Getting sufficient and high-quality sleep can be challenging for some, and it takes individualized care to access rejuvenating rest.

Best Practices:

- Reduce bright and blue-light exposure before bed. Exposure to light reduces melatonin in the brain and affects the circadian rhythm, so set aside the phone and turn the lights down before sleeping.
- Find a rhythm. Although maintaining a sleep schedule can be difficult as an athlete, a consistent sleep pattern supports circadian rhythm and melatonin levels. Prioritize your regular sleep schedule and supplement with short naps instead of late sleep-ins.
- Supplements. Melatonin (a key sleep hormone), magnesium (mineral with many demonstrated positive effects on sleep), jujube, PharmaGABA, and lavender aromatherapy are a few options.

- Maintain a sleep-conducive bedroom environment. Key factors that positively impact sleep are: cooler temperatures, darkness, little to no noise, and comfortable bed materials.
- Bring your own pillow if it means optimal rest.

Nutrition:

Proper nutrition is essential to achieving your highest level of athletic performance. Most athletes connect that they only feel as good as the food they've eaten before, during, and after training or competition. A targeted nutrition plan will give you the best chance of achieving your full potential. The easiest way to give your body all the energy and nutrients it needs, and the added benefit of self-confidence, is to eat a well-balanced and varied diet. A general plan is as follows, unless you require a specific diet for particular allergies or other individual needs:

Best Practices:

- All athletes know that carbohydrates are good for them. Carbs provide the energy source that muscles prefer during exercise. About 45 to 65% of our diet should come from carbs. Consume carbs at least 3-4 hours prior to workout to maximize energy, and consume them within 30 minutes to 4 hours after a workout to help restore glycogen stores. Foods such as potatoes, whole grain pasta, rice, bread, couscous, cereal, and other whole grains are basic carbs. Gluten-free diets may be necessary when celiac disease is involved or inflammation markers are high.
- Fat is a vital nutrient and plays a critical role in a wide number of bodily functions. Fat aids in the absorption of vitamins and protects our vital organs with padding. Fat is essential to maintain and improve endurance. Eating foods that contain fat is a great way to meet your energy needs

and perform. As we optimize training and intensify performance activity, we burn both carbs and fat, which need to be replenished. The more fat you have to draw on, the longer you can exercise before getting tired. Whole milk dairy products, organic olive or coconut oils, seeds, nuts, olives, avocados, and fatty fish are great sources of fat.

- Proteins aid in muscle synthesis and repair. Athletes need 1.2–2.0 grams of protein per kilogram of body weight. Seafood, meats, eggs, nuts, dairy, dark green vegetables, and legumes are excellent sources of protein.
- Vitamins and minerals are micronutrients that are needed in many processes throughout the body, especially for athletes. Eating nutrient-dense foods is the best way to get vitamins and minerals. This means foods with lots of colors (fruits and vegetables), whole grains, nuts, seeds, and a variety of lean protein sources (including

some vegetable sources of protein, such as beans). Choose nutrient-dense food 80% of the time, and leave 20% of food choices for fun. Eat a variety of foods, eat produce that is in-season, and eat fortified foods like nutritional shakes and bars.

- A word on salt. Sodium is one of the most important electrolytes in the human body. It controls the function of every cell in our body. Sodium (salt) plays an important role in fluid balance. Too much salt is not advisable as it can raise blood pressure. There are many sources of sodium including a wide range of grinds of salt (sea salt or Himalayan), soy sauce, and liquid amino acids.
- Finally, support the adrenal glands. Adrenal health is a lesser-known, but essential aspect of optimal body function for athletes. The adrenal glands produce hormones that regulate the immune system, metabolism, blood pressure, stress, and other key

functions. The physical stress of overtraining may deplete hormones produced by the adrenal glands. Overtraining can be done in a healthy way, but chronic overtraining can lead to serious health issues, including adrenal exhaustion and failure. Athletes must take heed to depletion; it's dangerous and possibly fatal. To support your adrenal health, prioritize rest, recovery, and proper nutrition. B vitamins and magnesium support adrenal health, as well as reducing intake of caffeine and sugar.

MENTAL HEALTH

The key to athletic performance is finding the balance between athletic drive, emotional well-being, and the passion to thrive.

For an athlete, a positive and determined mindset is a major asset to being a champion in sport and in life. **Technical skills and physical talent are only a part of the game; the other**

part is the mental side of engaging with the sport's demands. The advantages of developing laser-beam focus, a positive attitude, and the unique ability to carry the weight of positive and negative stresses distinguishes athletes as special people who exude spirited life-momentum. But over time, stresses can become dark forces pushing against one's passion and excellence in sport. The constant physical, psychological, and emotional output that equates to stress is universal for athletes but can become draining. Stresses ranging from nervous excitement or the abundance of attention from family, friends, and the outside world; your own inner critic or nerves displayed by coaches, family, teammates, and the media; or devastation over a performance setback or unfortunate injury can deplete the adrenals. Stress also plays a role in individual biorhythms, and from intensive training, there are direct affects on biochemistry, hormones, and moods.

For this reason, prioritizing rest, medication, cross training, smart nutrition and hydration, and micronutrients or supplements into daily life will support and also elevate mental and overall well-being.

Optimal mental health requires a hefty support system. This can mean family, friends, teammates, a therapist, a sports psychologist, and others. Sharing and discussing stressors and feelings is a necessary relief for mental well-being. We need to allow ourselves to accept the support of others. Athletes are known for mental fortification and durability, but sometimes we need help and treatment for our mental health—just as we may seek care for our physical health.

Optimal mental health also requires self-compassion amidst an insatiable drive to champion one's sport. Athletes at a high caliber will bode well with a regular practice of self-love, confidence, and positive self-talk. As a sports psychologist, I created a special technique to enhance self-awareness, intention, motivation, and momentum. It's called GAME F.A.C.E. and the goal is to encourage people to have fun while being serious about a goal. GAME F.A.C.E. sometimes causes an explosion of excitement and all-new purpose.

To play, choose your name or a keyword, then use the letters of the word to create a motivational phrase. For race-day or everyday winning in life, we choose GAME **F.A.C.E.** as an acronym for:

F is for Fun!

A is for Ambitious!

C is for Consistent!

E is for Excellence or Endure!

On race-day, we turn **R.A.C.E.** into:

Ready!

Ambitious!

Crush it!

Excellence!

Or if you want to embrace being a **Whole Athlete**, try:

W is for wellness and wholeness.

H is for helping myself, others, and the planet today and every day.

O is for opportunities to use my platform for a better world.

L is for love for self, others, and the planet.

E is for encouraging everyone to do their part to make the world a better place.

Paul, an athlete who struggled with self-esteem, soon thrived by using his name as the perfect acronym for self-affirmation:

P for Perfect as I am.

A for Ambitious Animal.

U for Unstoppable.

L for Lots of Love / Laugh at Self.

GAME F.A.C.E. not only energizes purpose and performance, it provides solutions.

> “
>
> **Be the best version of yourself in anthing that you do.**
>
> – Steph Curry
>
> ”

SOCIAL RESPONSIBILITY

CARING FOR HUMANITY AND OTHERS IN THE WORLD

SOCIAL RESPONSIBILITY

LOOKS LIKE THIS

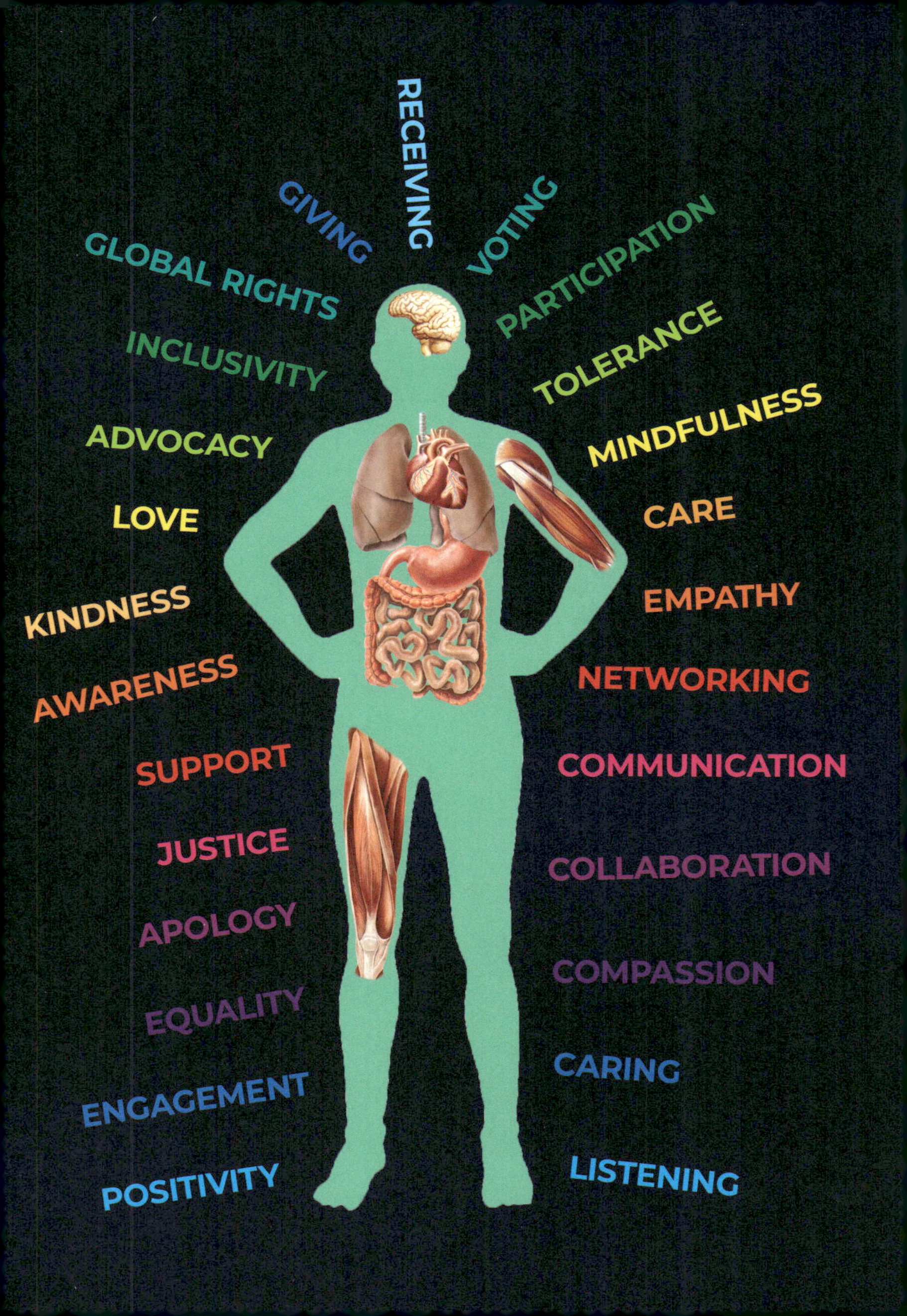

RECEIVING
GIVING
VOTING
GLOBAL RIGHTS
PARTICIPATION
INCLUSIVITY
TOLERANCE
ADVOCACY
MINDFULNESS
LOVE
CARE
KINDNESS
EMPATHY
AWARENESS
NETWORKING
SUPPORT
COMMUNICATION
JUSTICE
COLLABORATION
APOLOGY
COMPASSION
EQUALITY
CARING
ENGAGEMENT
POSITIVITY
LISTENING

SOCIAL RESPONSIBILITY IS THE SECOND pillar of embodying the values and lifestyle of a Whole Athlete. It means shifting your lens of focus from "self" to "whole," or caring for the greater good while you also care about your achievement in sport. Social responsibility is possessing awareness and understanding that global challenges affect humanity and society and that you will contribute to a specific cause to the best of your ability.

As an athlete, you are understandably concerned with your personal needs. It takes an exceptional amount of motivation and ambition to be an elite athlete, and these qualities can cause us to turn inward, away from the outstanding issues facing people close by or the global challenges facing humanity and the environment. Today, every serious athlete can choose to allocate some energy, awareness, life force, purpose, and commitment to inspire best practices for the benefit of a better world. There isn't anyone more empowered or able to influence great positive change.

Athletes. **We are natural role models.** Sports are pervasively popular within most cultures, and athletes command unique attention and influence. Athletes have the opportunity to lead by example, enact change by making conscious choices, and shift the tides of society. Athletes can use their unique circumstances and abilities to best impact and influence the world. A Whole Athlete not only strives to live as a role model for others, but accepts responsibility to encourage positive role models and mentors for others who need encouragement. It's one thing to be a person who earns titles, trophies, and steps up to the podium and another thing to be someone who steps up to help the greater whole.

Be unafraid to leverage your platform to speak out for multiple causes that touch your heart and life. Igniting change is only possible when we practice social responsibility and be a role model:

- Be informed: Read newspapers, connect to online media, and listen to public radio stations to be aware of current events in the world.
- Act responsibly: Practice responsibility in all areas of your life, and demonstrate care with yourself, your sport, your community, and the environment.
- Use your platform for advocacy: Identify a cause that resonates with you and speak up about it.
- Dedicate time or money to a cause: Turn your passion into a contribution, whether monetary or time or in-kind.

Identify a cause(s) that aligns with your values, galvanizes and inspires your passion, and provides an opportunity for impact. Impact happens when we embrace “one person, one cause, one day at a time” as our guide.

> **Unless someone like you cares a whole awful lot, nothing is going to get better. It’s not.**
>
> – Dr. Seuss

ENVIRONMENTAL RESPONSIBILITY

CARING FOR EARTH'S BIODIVERSITY

ENVIRONMENTAL RESPONSIBILITY

LOOKS LIKE THIS

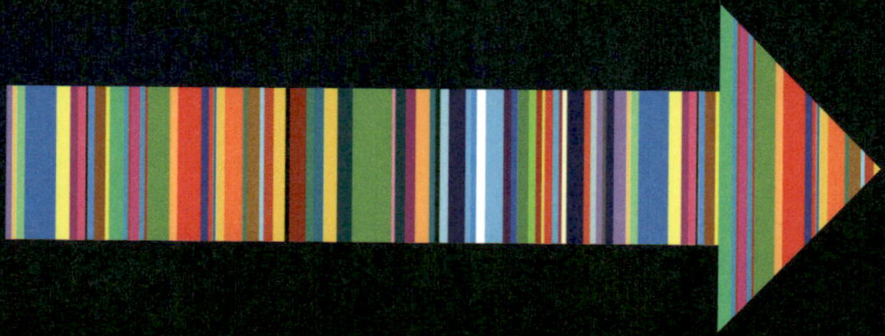

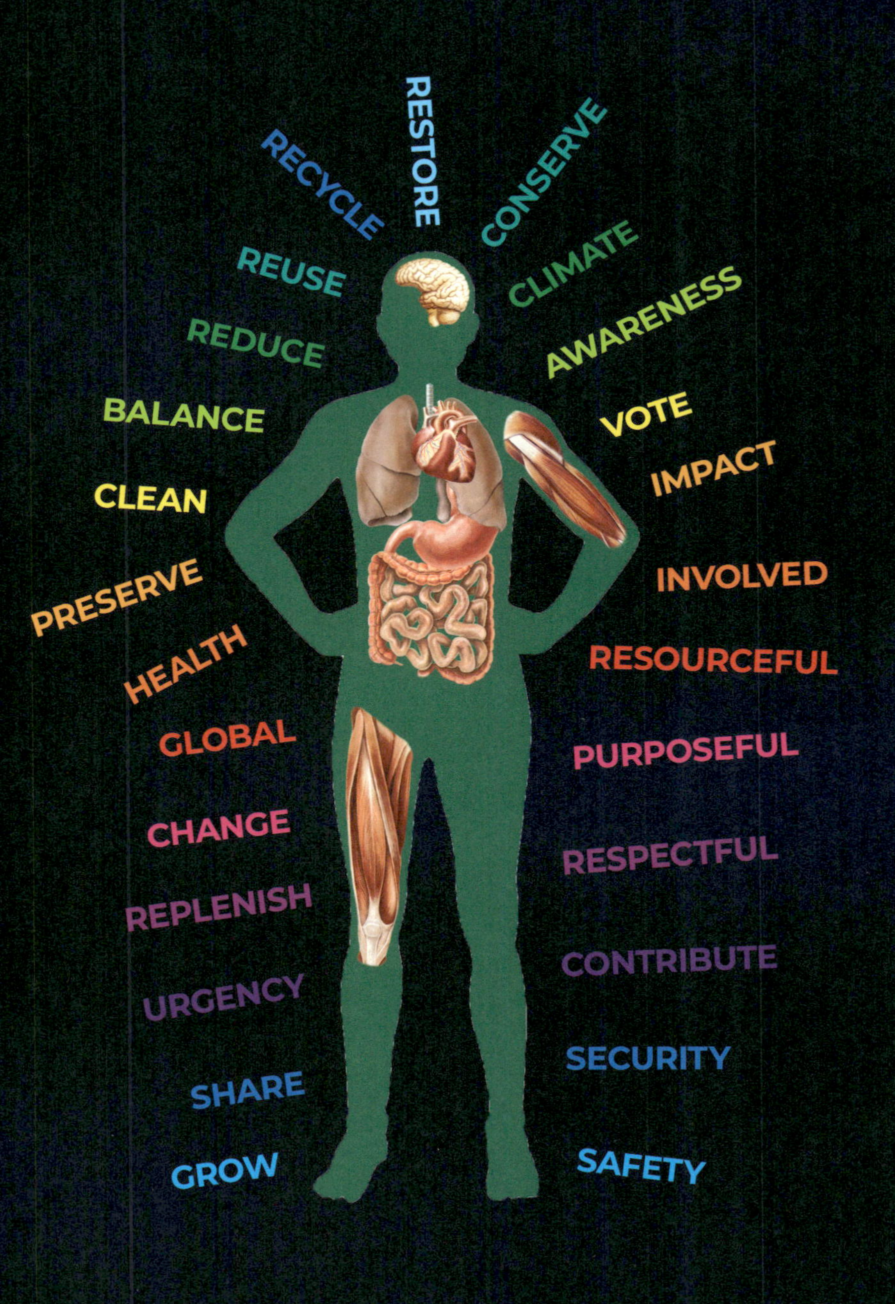
RESTORE
RECYCLE
CONSERVE
REUSE
CLIMATE
REDUCE
AWARENESS
BALANCE
VOTE
IMPACT
CLEAN
INVOLVED
PRESERVE
HEALTH
RESOURCEFUL
GLOBAL
PURPOSEFUL
CHANGE
RESPECTFUL
REPLENISH
CONTRIBUTE
URGENCY
SECURITY
SHARE
GROW
SAFETY

OUR PLANET IS ON THE BRINK OF A severe environmental crisis making all of us vulnerable to existing and potential disasters. Environmental responsibility is choosing a lifestyle that includes ecologically-minded habits, taking care of the earth day-to-day, as well as taking action to enact greater systemic and cultural change. Neuroscientists tell us that hope actually helps to organize our brains toward solutions, so hope is power, and it's just the power we need now.

Eight billion humans inhabit the planet but the size of our population does not have to mean more emissions and more harm to our climate. Athletes have a unique relationship to the earth and a unique environmental impact. **Athletes and their fans generate a large carbon footprint.** The circumstances of practicing/training, competing, traveling, and building venues for spectators all have distinct environmental impacts. Athletes have an exceptional duty to take environmental responsibility. We need to adjust our habits and lifestyle so that they are supportive of our earth. We can also champion change from everyone in this area.

The most effective way to help reduce global emissions is a conscious change in lifestyle. Research shows that most people have an incorrect impression of what actions actually make a difference in terms of their environmental impact. People tend to underestimate the positive impact of actions that are a little more challenging, such as veganism, and overestimate the positive impact of simpler actions like recycling. The actions that result in the greatest reduction of personal greenhouse gas emissions include living car-free, using renewable electricity, avoiding air travel, and eating a vegan diet. Vegetarianism, eating organic, and installing heat pumps have moderate effects, while recycling, carpooling, and using energy-efficient appliances have very minimal impacts on personal greenhouse gas emissions. Misinformation about the relative impact of these actions has been widely spread, and it means that people often focus on menial tasks when they could more greatly reduce their emissions through a lifestyle change.

As role models, athletes can take these tangible steps to reflect their commitment to environmental responsibility:

EAT FOR PERFORMANCE AND FOR THE PLANET

Food is powerful. Every day, our unique food choices fuel our bodies, bring us closer to others, and connect us to nature. Our eating choices have great social and environmental impact. It is undeniable that a plant-centered diet is better for our planet and our health, but how can athletes meet their unique physical needs while still caring for the planet?

The primary way to eat for the planet is through reducing our consumption of animal products like meat and dairy. The livestock and dairy industries consume massive amounts of water, land, grain, and fossil fuels, and contribute strongly to global emissions, causing extreme detriment to the environment.

According to the Mayo Clinic, "people who eat red meat are at an increased risk of death from heart disease, stroke, or diabetes," and "processed meats also increase the risk of death from these diseases." So, by reducing our consumption of animal products, we can care for ourselves in addition to the planet.

For athletes, this means finding alternative sources of protein, such as seitan, beans and rice, tofu, lentils, and other plant-based proteins. If you do eat meat, ensure that it is sourced sustainably, and try to choose chicken and sustainable fish over red meat.

Another way to eat for the planet is to eat seasonal and local produce. Eating seasonal and local produce equates to fewer greenhouse gas emissions, because your food undergoes less travel and processing.

Finally, work to avoid excess food packaging and consider buying in bulk. Pre-packaged foods are a huge source of plastic waste, and buying in bulk reduces this waste. Bring your own reusable bags or containers and purchase only what you need.

TRAVEL MORE SUSTAINABLY

Reduce flying as much as possible; optimize travel itineraries to cut down on travel and utilize other forms of transportation, like trains and buses. When you need to fly, consider using a carbon offset. Carbon offsetting works to reduce CO_2 in the atmosphere primarily through forestry projects (planting trees to sequester carbon from the atmosphere) and energy projects (reducing energy sources reliant on fossil fuels). Some airlines offer carbon offset when booking a flight, but you can also use nonprofits to offset your flights. There is a section in the index of organizations at the end of this book covering carbon offset.

ALIGN WITH CLIMATE-RESPONSIBLE PARTNERS

Collaborating with a few well-chosen sustainable organizations benefits both the environment and the athlete. As an athlete, you can help partners achieve their sustainability goals through accountability and inspiration. You can collaborate on climate and sustainability projects to improve the environmental impact of the organization and to champion global change.

Before partnering with an organization, do your research. Ensure that they not only promote sustainability but act on it. The index of organizations at this book's end includes many sustainable organizations.

USE YOUR PLATFORM TO INSTIGATE POSITIVE ENVIRONMENTAL CHANGE

Your platform is a perfect stepping-point for powerful change. Use your social media channels to join or start campaigns for sustainable awareness and action, share and advocate for sustainable habits, and elevate the voices and messages of those championing change. In addition, many communities and groups support athletes in advocacy. Working with these connections can amplify positive environmental transformation.

REDUCE WASTE PRODUCTION

A significant part of our environmental impact is our production of waste, including plastics, disposables, trash, and more. Making small changes in your day-to-day life can greatly reduce both your waste production and your environmental impact.

First, always compost and recycle when possible. Properly sorting waste means less ends up in landfills.

Donate, share, or resell unwanted and unworn clothing. Avoid fast-fashion brands and try to purchase from sustainable clothing brands, some of which are listed in the index of organizations at the end of this book.

Consider using a greywater system in your home. Greywater systems redirect and recycle the water used for washing (laundry, bathing, handwashing, etc.) for a second purpose, like irrigation or flushing toilets. Greywater systems both conserve water and reduce utilities costs.

Replace single-use items with reusables, such as bringing your own travel mug to a coffee shop and using metal straws, cloth napkins, and reusable containers, whenever possible.

CHOOSE CONSCIOUS BRANDS

Sustainable clothing and toiletries brands are available widely and many support causes that care for the earth and its inhabitants.

And when you are in the market for appliances, buy ones that use less energy and water and create less food spoilage. These will also save you money over their years of use. The index of organizations at the end of this book lists many sustainable options for brands.

“

What makes something special is not just what you have to gain, but what you feel there is to lose.

– Andre Agassi

”

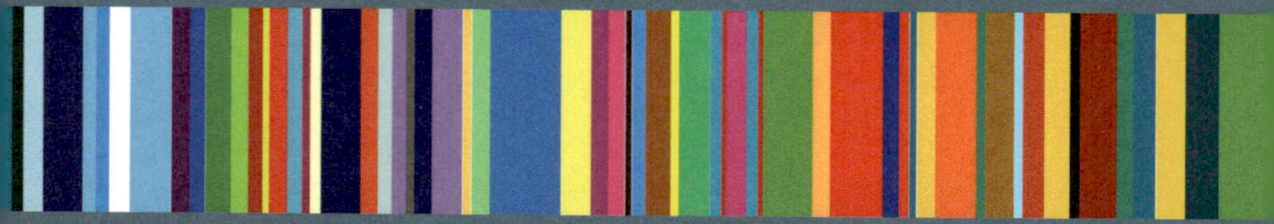

WHOLE ATHLETE

CONTRIBUTING TO A BETTER WORLD

A WHOLE ATHLETE

LOOKS LIKE THIS

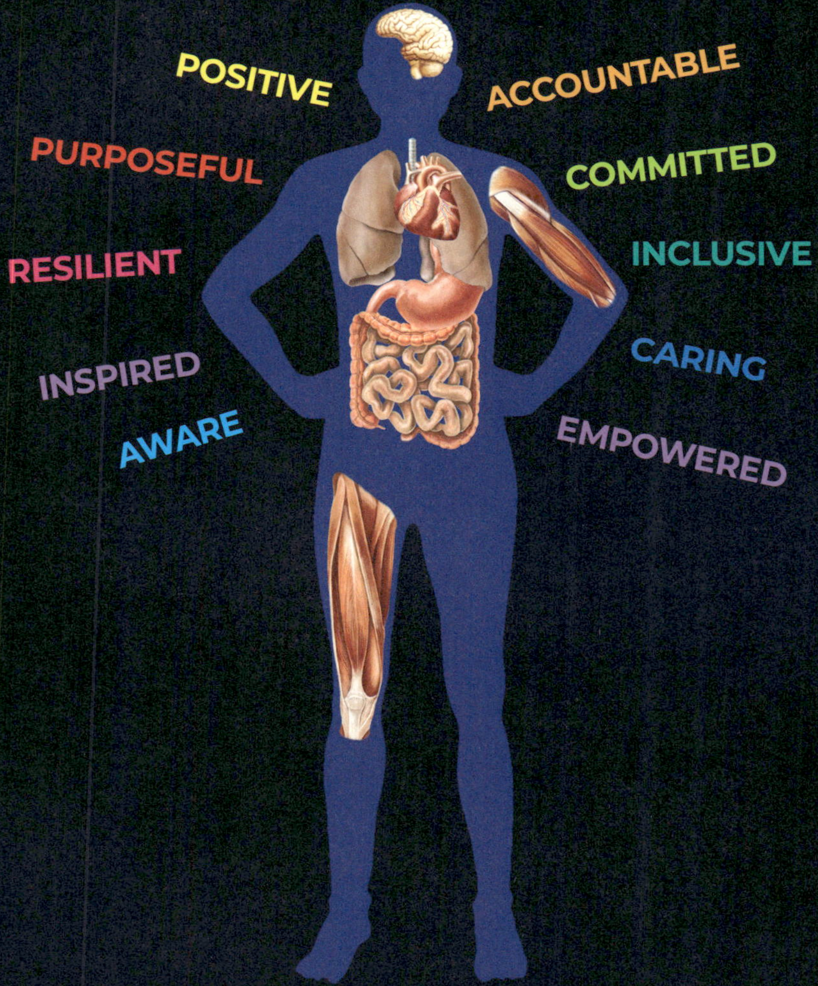
POSITIVE
ACCOUNTABLE
PURPOSEFUL
COMMITTED
RESILIENT
INCLUSIVE
INSPIRED
CARING
AWARE
EMPOWERED

HOW TO CHAMPIO

ONE PERSON • ONE CA

HEALTHY COMMUNITY

A C T I O N S

- Exercise daily and choose human powered transportation whenever possible.
- Give more than you take.
- Behave as a role model.
- Encourage and celebrate others' achievements.
- Be accountable at home, work, and school.
- Turn off vehicle engine when parked.
- Pick up litter, organize clean-ups.
- Eat nutritiously.
- Shop Fair Trade products and at farmer's markets.
- Learn basic First Aid and CPR.
- Ask local restaurants and dry cleaners to avoid toxic cleaning products and plastics.
- Consider a drought resistant garden.
- Initiate community-wide health events, such as blood donation, food and clothing drives, health fairs, and sports competitions.
- Support and host charitable events for local issues such as hunger, homelessness, mental illness, socia injustice, catastrophic events, and water pollution.

CHOOSE TO DO ONE ACTION EVEF
THE COMMUNIT

BE TH

OSITIVE CHANGE

E • ONE DAY AT A TIME

HEALTHY PLANET

Walk, bike, skateboard, or carpool to work, school, errands, and social events.

Commit to 100% ecological household papers and soaps; no aerosols, plastics, perfumes or dyes.

Re-use glass jars and containers for warm and cold drinks and food storage.

Turn off lights, water, appliances, and technology products when not needed.

Limit laundry and dishwasher cycles; use cold water and shortest settings.

Reduce heat consumption at home, office, and school by wearing warm clothing.

Consume fewer material things. Upcycle or donate possessions.

Organize paperless billing, online banking, news, and magazine subscriptions.

Reject harmful pesticides.

Avoid air travel or buy carbon offsets when you fly.

Donate to organizations focused on clean air, water, and land; energy conservation; climate change; poverty; and war relief.

AY THAT BETTERS YOUR SELF,
ND THE PLANET.

HANGE.

BY EMBRACING YOUR ROLE AS AN influencer and Whole Athlete, you are globally responsible for caring for yourself, others, and the environment thereby igniting global change–**one person, one cause, one day at a time.**

YOU, as an athlete, have been given a monumental opportunity to make a difference for the world. With the unique attention, circumstances, and respect that society has for athletes, you possess the platform to encourage and inspire others to take responsibility and action for a better world. You can now show the world how a Whole Athlete makes the whole world better.

- **A Whole Athlete champions positive activity and inspires everyone around them to do the same.**
- **A Whole Athlete shares their journey with others and acts with compassion and generosity to help those in need.**

- A Whole Athlete uses their platform not just to benefit themselves, but also to champion other people and the environment.
- A Whole Athlete inspires their family, community, and culture to become whole, too.

WHOLE ATHLETE PLEDGE

I recognize that our world requires a monumental shift and that I can be an athlete who steps up to make a difference. I understand the time is now to champion the well-being of myself, other people, and the whole planet.

I PLEDGE TO DO MY BEST TO MAKE A DIFFERENCE!

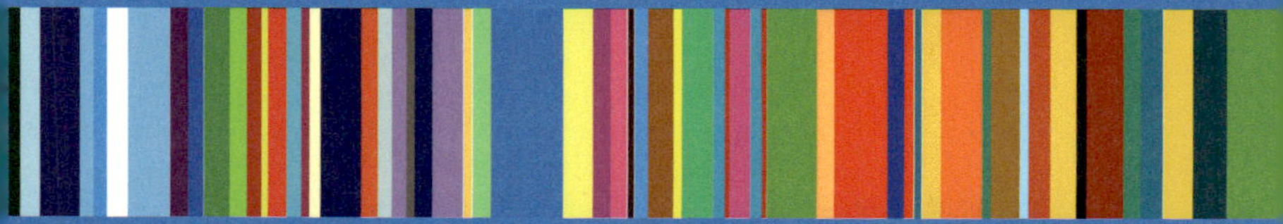

AFTERWORD

Thank you for considering using the enormous potential you posess as an athlete, a role model, and a leader to contribute to a better world.

Let's do more with all that we have. Let's come together to help people and other living things in need. Let's be conscious, connected, and active every day.

To learn more or get involved visit wholechampion.org or email info@wholechampion.org.

“

Seek wisdom from nature.
Live in truth.
Give more than you take.
Love deeply.
Say thank you.
Begin again.

– Barbara Edelston Peterson

”

RESOURCES

SUSTAINABLE ORGANIZATIONS AND NONPROFITS

BRAND	MISSION
350.org	Widespread member organization utilizes campaigns and grassroots organizing to oppose fossil fuel projects, support clean energy, and build an equitable zero-carbon economy.
5 Gyres Institute	Inspires individual and organizational changes to address plastic pollution
American Forests	Conservational organization to restore, protect, and expand forests and forest policy
Cool Effect	Works to reduce carbon emissions in a variety of ways
Earthjustice	Environmental law organization
Eden Projects	Nonprofit working to employ people through reforestation
Fashion Revolution	Global movement motivating towards a sustainable fashion industry
Fibershed	Works to create sustainable fiber systems for earth-friendly textiles and clothing
Lonely Whale Foundation	Protects and restores oceans through collaboration, inspiration, and the support of collective action, ideas, and campaigns
Oceane	International organization that protects and restores the oceans
1% for the Planet	Global network for nonprofits, businesses, and individuals to unite for an environmentally healthy world
One Tree Planted	Nonprofit that plants a tree for every dollar donated with the help of Tree Ambassadors

Rainforest Action Network	Works to preserve forests, the climate, and human rights by taking action against corporations and industries enabling climate change and deforestation.
Sierra Club	Grassroots environmental organization working to protect nature and increase access to it.
The Jane Goodall Institute	Nature conservation focused on wildlife, action through education and inspiration
The Soil Association	Promotes and facilitates regenerative agriculture
Wild Earth Allies	Works with local organizations and individuals to support biodiversity and wildlife

SUSTAINABLE SPORTING GEAR

BRAND	MISSION
EarthHero	Certified B Corp, 1% For the Planet member, Climate Neutral certified, zero waste, sustainable and eco-friendly materials
Eco Sports	Sustainable sporting equipment made from TPU (biodegradable, recyclable, vegan), plastic-free packaging, 10% of profits donated towards planting trees
Trek Bicycles	Uses recycled and reclaimed materials, renewable energy, lots of recyclable packaging, working to protect and establish bike trails, reduce environmental impact
Waboba	REWILD Eco-Friendly Series made from sustainable materials, recycled packaging
Yama Mountain Gear	1% For the Planet member, carbon neutral via carbon offsets, renewable energy, some recycled materials, some recycled packaging, transparency

SUSTAINABLE CLOTHING BRANDS

BRAND	MISSION
ABLE	Certified B Corp., feminist brand creating economic opportunities for women to provide for themselves
Allbirds	Shoes made from eco-friendly, sustainable, and recycled materials
Back Beat Co.	Primarily USA-manufactured, certified organic cotton, eco-friendly materials, recycled packaging
Cariuma	Eco-friendly materials, and plants two trees in the Brazilian rainforest for every pair of shoes purchased
Cotopaxi	Uses recycled materials and facilitates sustainable and fair working conditions
Eileen Fisher	Certified B Corp, Fair Trade Certified collections, circular and recycling initiatives
Everlane	Utilizes recycled materials, very transparent
Fair Indigo	Creates long lasting clothes, certified organic, fair wages, gives back to the community
Girlfriend Collective	100% recyclable packaging, eco-friendly materials made from wasted materials
Kotn	Certified B Corp., certified organic cotton, works to promote and facilitate safe in fair labor standards, Gives back to Egyptian communities
MATE The Label	Climate neutral, organic and non-toxic materials, gives back to environmental causes
Naadam	Almost all materials are renewable or recycled, compensates material sources fairly
Outerknown	Fibers are 90% organic, recycle, or regenerated
Pact	Fair trade certified, certified organic cotton, carbon offset for shipping, recyclable packaging, makes cotton basics

Patagonia	Fair trade certified factories, materials are mostly sustainable
Picture Organic Clothing	Certified B Corp, Fair Wear Foundation member, climate action initiatives, very transparent, many eco-friendly materials
PrAna	Fair trade certified, extremely transparent and sustainable, yoga and outdoor clothing
Purusha People	Plastic-free, eco-friendly materials, non-toxic dyes, local manufacturing
Quince	Sustainable and organic materials, recycle plastics, certified ethical production, sustainability "as the standard, not a luxury "
Reformation	Climate neutral certified, sustainable fabrics, safe and fair working conditions, living wages
Summersalt	Sustainable swimwear, as leisure, and loungewear from eco-friendly factories and materials
Tentree	Sustainable materials, climate neutral certified, certified B corporation, 10 trees planted for every item purchased
United By Blue	Eco-friendly outdoor clothing, 1 pound of trash removed from oceans and waterways for each item sold

SUSTAINABLE KITCHEN/BATH BRANDS

BRAND	MISSION
Beko	Sustainable home appliances, working to reduce greenhouse gas emissions and energy consumption, recycles water during manufacturing, uniquely sustainable products
Blueland	Refillable cleaning products; starter kit comes with a "forever bottle" where are you mix tablets with water, you can order refill tablets

Bosch	Climate neutral, environmentally friendly appliances that are all energy star certified, working to increase renewable energy use, reduce water used, and improve circularity
Cleancult	Nontoxic, zero Waste, plant-based cleaning products With 100% recyclable packaging, carbon neutral shipments
EVO	Products made from Wood Plastic Composite; more eco-friendly plastic alternative
Miele	Eco-friendly appliances, working to become carbon neutral, most appliances meet the highest energy efficiency category
Nebia	Water saving shower heads and PVC free shower curtains
One Planet	Sustainable and reusable products, plastic-free alternatives
Pur Home	Natural, plant-based, biodegradable, safe household cleaning products, ethically sourced ingredients
Seventh Generation	Certified B Corp, working towards 100% zero-waste and 100% renewable energy, some biodegradable products
Simple Green	All-purpose environmentally-friendly cleaner and degreaser
SMEG	eco-friendly home appliances that utilize high performance with low energy consumption, most appliances meet the highest energy efficiency class rating, recyclable materials prioritized
Who Gives a Crap	Eco-friendly, 100% recycled fiber toilet paper

SUSTAINABLE TOILETRIES BRANDS

BRAND	MISSION
Dab Herb	Plastic free beauty brand with skin care and zero-waste make up, refill options
Dr. Bronners	Certified organic, nearly zero-waste, renewable energy systems, ethical sourcing, recyclable materials, Fair Trade projects, natural ingredients, charity work
Dermatone	Sunscreen that is reef-safe and contains natural ingredients. Some products are water-free
Dirty Hippie	Zero waste, organic, fully plant or mineral based
EcoRoots	Waste free beauty and skin care products, zero waste beauty tools
EmpireSquid Organics	Zero waste skin care, all natural ingredients, no palm oil
EO Products	Plant-based body care products incorporating organic and sustainable essential oils
Ethique	Sustainable packaging, 08 shampoos and conditioners, 100% plastic free, natural products, Palm oil free
Everyday Humans	Sunscreen company that has Plastic Neutral and Climate Neutral certifications, recycled and recyclable packaging, animal testing free, 1% for the Planet member
Fat & the Moon	Handmade to order, natural and ethically harvested ingredients
Meow Meow Tweet	Eco-friendly skin care, many zero waste products and sustainable practices and materials
Prose	Customizable hair care that is certified climate neutral, certified B Corporation
Skinnies	Uses sugar cane packaging and uses smaller packaging to reduce carbon footprint, plus product contains no water.

Sonrei	Refillable packaging and member of 1% for the Planet
Trestique	Zero waste makeup, refillable beauty products, mostly natural ingredients

CARBON OFFSET RESOURCES

BRAND	MISSION
Atmosfair	Focus on offsetting the environmental impact of air travel, projects in many countries working to promote sustainable travel and sustainable energy
CarbonPay	Offers payment cards that automatically offset carbon footprints, simplifies everyday climate action
Clear	Supports very high quality projects, all carbon offsets are certified by the quality assurance standard for carbon offsetting, very precise carbon offset calculator
Myclimate	Easy to use carbon offset calculator, provides resources for reducing carbon footprint
Native Energy	Long running organization, certified B Corp., very transparent, calculator available, variety of projects
Sustainable Travel International	Works to minimize the negative effects of tourism and protect tourist destinations, carbon footprint calculator, projects focused on forest and biodiversity, clean and efficient energy, blue carbon, aid for local communities
TerraPass	Carbon calculator, investments help fund energy efficiency, sustainable farming, other environmental projects

Brands change, go out of business, merge with other companies, are acquired or sold. These lists are not exhaustive but are what we created at the time of publication.

GLOSSARY

WHOLE ATHLETE GLOSSARY

ACCOUNTABILITY: Holding yourself to the truth, your word, promise, or commitment.

AUTHENTICITY: Being true to yourself by acting according to your personal values. Applying your unique internal vision to the external world.

AWARENESS: Consciousness, or knowledge of existence, is like light—it illuminates a situation or state of mind. From this springs awareness (knowing the difference between right and wrong). A whole champion's awareness motivates them to fight wrong in the world, and to work for well-being on a personal, local, and global scale.

CARE: Attention to providing what's necessary for the health, welfare, maintenance, and protection of others. Care is taking time to complete something correctly and a focus on avoiding needless damage or risk.

CHAMPION: A champion stands up for a cause and sees it through to completion. To champion a sport, a cause, or an ideology, you need to be an unstoppable force until your goal is achieved. A whole champion is driven to achieve, and is unrelenting in accomplishing good for humanity and the environment, not just the self. A whole champion leverages their achievements and most compelling ideas to support the greater good.

KINDNESS: The quality of being friendly, generous, and considerate. Kindness is the foundation for making positive, whole change.

ENVIRONMENTAL RESPONSIBILITY: A conscious mindset that the planet needs care, protection, recovery, and an opportunity to flourish in its natural state. Embrace a lifestyle that nourishes and champions the environment.

Purposeful effort to do one's part for planet Earth:

Minimize your ecological footprint through sustainable, recyclable, "green" practices and products that protect Mother Nature. Treat the environment the way you would a family member or a friend.

INCLUSIVITY: An open attitude welcoming all people, regardless of age, gender, race, ethnicity, religion, socioeconomic background, or geographic location. Inclusivity means practicing open-mindedness, respect, tolerance, social justice, and love for other human beings.

MOTIVATION: An inner force that moves you physically, mentally, and spiritually. It can come from a voice in your head, emotion in your heart, or drive in your gut to do the right thing.

NETWORK: A system or group of people. If we zoom out, we can see that through interconnectivity, everything around us is potentially a network that can be used in positive ways to improve the world.

PERSONAL RESPONSIBILITY: Caring for oneself by holding oneself accountable. It's self-love, self-care, and self-work—an investment in personal development. It's awareness and balance of mind, body, and spirit. Personal responsibility leads to the pride and empowerment that result from doing one's best.

RESPONSIBILITY: A decision to start thinking, feeling, and acting with awareness and intention. It is a conscious effort to do the right thing, in large or small ways, for the greater good.

SELF-CARE: Kindness, acceptance, and confidence in yourself throughout life. Understanding your unique qualities and characteristics. Practicing self-care means becoming a champion of yourself through love, compassion, patience, and authentic, passionate pursuits.

SOCIAL RESPONSIBILITY: Caring for oneself and others; taking action to benefit other people. Awareness, compassion, and action—social responsibility means giving more than you take. It could be as simple as offering to carry someone's groceries, or as involved as participating in a food drop to a village stricken by natural disaster or war. It can manifest as organizing a peaceful march to benefit a worthy cause.

UPCYCLING: A form of creative recycling centered around reusing items in your everyday life to decrease your ecological footprint.

WHOLE A state of harmony, completion, or resolution ultimately achieved by a group effort that begins with a single person. Wholeness means practicing awareness, responsibility, and taking action for a better world. It'a taking personal, social, and environmental responsibility for the planet.

ENVIRONMENTAL GLOSSARY

ALTERNATIVE ENERGY	Energy created using methods that don't deplete natural resources or cause harm to the environment; these avoid using fossil fuels and nuclear power.
BIODEGRADABLE	Something capable of decomposing into its basic components.
BIODIESEL	A renewable fuel for diesel engines derived from natural oils.
BIOMASS	Organic matter that can be used as a fuel, usually to generate electricity.
BLACKWATER	Blackwater is wastewater from toilets which can't be reused because of contamination.
CARBON EMISSIONS	Pollution released into the atmosphere from carbon dioxide and carbon monoxide, produced by motor vehicles, planes, and manufacturing.
CARBON FOOTPRINT	The amount of carbon dioxide, in tons, produced by an individual or an organization; can be affected by lifestyle and practices.

CARBON NEGATIVE Exceeding carbon neutrality by removing additional carbon dioxide from the atmosphere beyond what one produces; also referred to as carbon negative.

CARBON NEUTRAL When an individual or organization has net-zero carbon emissions, often through using carbon offset.

CARBON OFFSET A credit that a person or organization can purchase to compensate for its carbon footprint; carbon neutral is achieved when carbon offsets purchased are equivalent to the amount of carbon produced.

CARBON SEQUESTRATION Capturing and storing carbon to prevent it from staying in the atmosphere; can be through natural ways like planting a tree or manufactured.

CARBON SINKS A carbon sink is anything that absorbs more carbon from the atmosphere than it releases, like plants, the ocean, and soil.

CIRCULAR ECONOMY A system designed to eliminate waste by reusing, sharing, repairing, and recycling resources, in contrast to a linear system, where the cycle is to make, use, and dispose.

CLIMATE CHANGE Climate change refers to long-term shifts in temperatures and weather patterns. Human activities have been the main driver of long-term climate change, primarily due to burning fossil fuels like coal, oil, and gas.

CLIMATE POSITIVE Exceeding carbon neutrality by removing additional carbon dioxide from the atmosphere beyond what one produces; also referred to as climate positive.

CLIMATE RESILIENCE Climate resilience is the ability to prepare for and respond to dangerous events or trends related to the climate. Improving climate resilience involves assessing the risks climate change poses and preparing ways to mediate or prevent these risks.

CLOSED-LOOP The term “closed-loop” applies to any system, like the economy or recycling where materials and resources are reused to create new products. A closed-loop system reduces waste production and use of natural resources.

COMPOSTING	Controlled decomposition of organic material.
CONSERVATION	The act of protecting the Earth's natural resources for current and future generations.
CRADLE TO CRADLE	Cradle to cradle refers to creating products that can be truly recycled, either by being reused or returned to the Earth through decomposition.
DEFORESTATION	Conversion of forested lands into non-forest use.
ECODISTRICTS	An ecodistrict is a community created to embody a holistically sustainable way of life.
ECO-CONSCIOUS	A mentality focused on reducing harm to the environment wherever possible.
ECO-FRIENDLY	Environmentally-minded actions that cause minimal harm to the earth.
ECOLOGICAL FOOTPRINT	Measurement based on the amount of nature it takes to support something.
ECOLOGICAL RESTORATION	The artificial process of restoring an ecosystem to its original form—

which is nearly impossible to fully repair—but it's still important to do as much as possible.

ENERGY EFFICIENT	Uses the smallest amount of energy possible to provide power.
FAIRTRADE	Principles of fair treatment, wages, and safe working conditions for workers.
GEOTHERMAL ENERGY	Renewable energy generated by heat coming from the Earth's core; typically hot steam or water heated from within the Earth.
GLOBAL WARMING	Global warming is the long-term heating of Earth's surface caused by human activities, primarily fossil fuel burning, which increases heat-trapping greenhouse gas levels in Earth's atmosphere.
GREEN BUILDING	Green building refers to using sustainable and environmentally-friendly materials and processes to build and maintain structures.
GREENHOUSE EFFECT	The process by which excessive heat is trapped in the atmosphere due to the build-up of greenhouse gases.
GREENWASHING	Misrepresenting something as being "green" when it's not

environmentally-friendly.

GREYWATER	The relatively clean wastewater from baths, sinks, laundry machines, and other kitchen appliances.
GREYWATER SYSTEM	This system filters greywater to remove impurities, allowing it be reused for watering plants and irrigation.
NAKED PACKAGING	Products that are sold without packaging.
NATURAL RESOURCES	Materials or substances such as minerals, forests, water, and fertile land that occur in nature.
NET-ZERO	Achieving a balance between emissions produced and emissions removed from the atmosphere; also known as carbon neutrality.
ORGANIC	Food and farming methods that don't use chemical fertilizers, pesticides, or other artificial agents.
POST-CONSUMER	Previously used by consumers before being reprocessed into a new product.

RAINWATER HARVESTING	Rainwater harvesting is the collection and storage of rainwater.
RECLAIMED	Waste materials refurbished for new products.
RECYCLING	To reprocess reusable goods.
REFORESTATION	Planting of forests on lands that have been depleted.
RENEWABLE ENERGY	Electricity from replenishable sources such as geothermal, hydropower, solar, and wind.
RENEWABLE RESOURCES	Renewable resources are an energy source that cannot be depleted and are able to supply a continuous source of clean energy, like the wind and sunlight.
SOLAR ENERGY	Any type of energy generated by the sun.
SUSTAINABILITY	Sustainability involves fulfilling the needs of current generations without compromising the needs of future generations, while ensuring a balance between economic growth, environmental care, and social well-being.

WATER SCARCITY A shortage of water to meet the needs of living organisms—caused by unequal access to water and excessive use of water among different social groups.

WATER SECURITY The state of having reliable access to a sufficient quantity of clean water.

WIND ENERGY Energy generated by wind turbines converting the kinetic energy in the wind to mechanical power.

WISH-CYCLING An aspirational approach to recycling items without knowing if they're recyclable but expecting them to be properly dealt with.

ZERO-WASTE Avoiding products that create waste by using tactics like buying in bulk and using reusable products.

SOURCES: https://sustainablereview.com/sustainability-101-terms-and-definitions/

https://www.architecturaldigest.com/story/go-green-glossary

Oxford Dictionary